KU-048-863

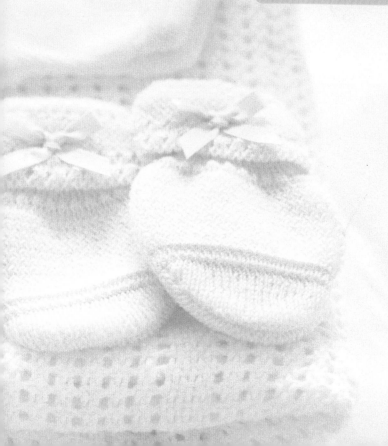

Pregnancy

ESSENTIALS

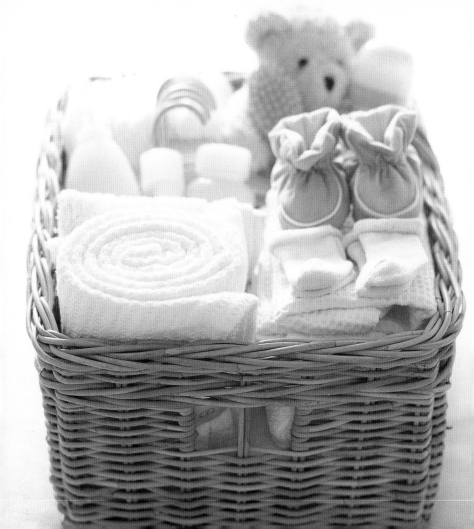

Pregnancy

ESSENTIALS

DR CAROL COOPER

RYLAND
PETERS
& SMALL

LONDON NEW YORK

SENIOR DESIGNER Liz Sephton
SENIOR EDITOR Henrietta Heald
PICTURE RESEARCHER Emily Westlake
PRODUCTION Gemma Moules
PUBLISHING DIRECTOR Alison Starling

First published in the UK in 2008
by Ryland Peters & Small
20–21 Jockey's Fields
London WC1R 4BW
www.rylandpeters.com

Text copyright © Carol Cooper 2008
Design and commissioned photographs
copyright © Ryland Peters & Small
Photographs copyright © Stockbyte
pages 21, 47, 52–53, 102

10 9 8 7 6 5 4 3 2 1

ISBN 978-1-84597-601-9

A CIP record for this book is available from
the British Library.

Printed and bound in China

Neither the author nor the publisher can be held
responsible for any claim arising from the use or
misuse of suggestions made in this book. While
every effort has been made to ensure that the
information contained in the book is accurate and
up to date, it is advisory only and should not be
used as an alternative to seeking specialist medical
advice. Consult your doctor if you are worried
about any health issue affecting you or your child.

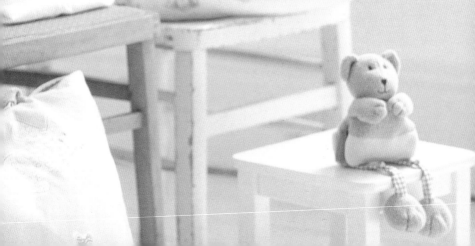

CONTENTS

INTRODUCTION

Expectant mothers (and fathers) want to know as much as they possibly can about their growing baby and about what happens at each stage of gestation. There are also many changes taking place in the woman's own body. Some of the developments are welcome, while others, such as piles, are a real nuisance and, frankly, have little to recommend them. Then there are problems such as rhesus disease and pre-eclampsia. While these may never happen during your pregnancy, it is still good to know something about them.

All in all, that makes a lot to pack into a short book. You'll find the essentials here in short snippets – ideal for the sagging powers of concentration that many mums-to-be complain about.

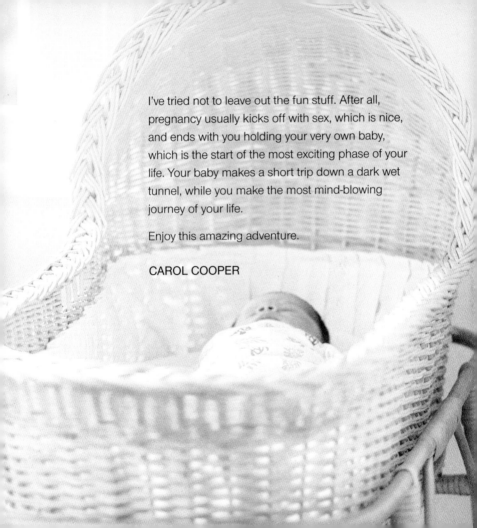

I've tried not to leave out the fun stuff. After all, pregnancy usually kicks off with sex, which is nice, and ends with you holding your very own baby, which is the start of the most exciting phase of your life. Your baby makes a short trip down a dark wet tunnel, while you make the most mind-blowing journey of your life.

Enjoy this amazing adventure.

CAROL COOPER

MAKING A GREAT START

A baby is the most intricate and most interesting thing anyone could possibly create. When you are building a baby, you have got to get the foundations right.

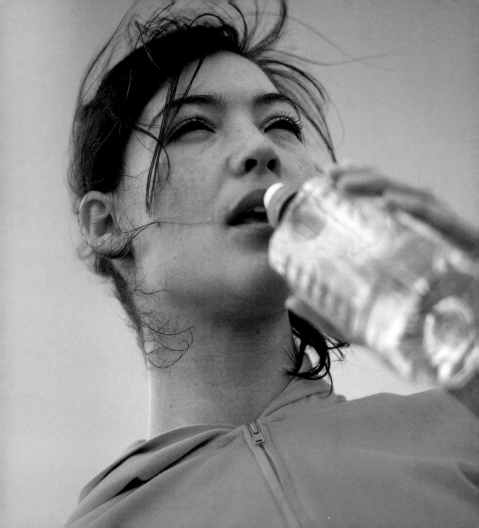

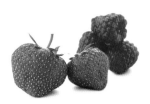

Over a period of eight and a half months (or 266 days) of gestation, one tiny cell turns into a small but complex human being. How the expectant mother lives in those formative months can make a big difference to the way her baby turns out.

food & drink

You needn't 'eat for two', but follow a **balanced diet**, with five helpings of **fruit and vegetables** a day, plenty of **protein** such as meat and fish, and ideally lots of **dairy products** – in addition to fibre, protein and vitamins (including folate), pregnant women need iron and calcium.

Carbohydrates are better eaten in the form of **complex carbohydrates** of the kind found in potatoes and wholemeal bread. Limit your intake of simple carbohydrates such as those in cakes and biscuits.

Low-fat foods are usually recommended for health, but your developing baby needs essential fatty acids, especially LCPUFAs (long-chain polyunsaturated fatty acids) for brain and eye development. You can get LCPUFAs in sunflower oil, evening primrose oil, oily fish and soya.

Although oily fish is good, bigger fish such as shark and tuna can be high in mercury, which may be toxic to your baby. Eat these less often, choosing instead **mackerel**, **herrings**, **sardines** and **pilchards**.

FOODS TO AVOID

- soft-ripened cheeses such as Brie, Camembert and blue cheeses: they can contain listeria, bacteria that are harmful to your baby

- paté and cook–chill foods (unless you've heated the chilled food very thoroughly): again, they may contain listeria

- raw or undercooked meats, unpasteurized dairy foods, unwashed vegetables or fruit: they can contain the parasite toxoplasma, which carries a risk of miscarriage and birth defects; rare meat contains *E. coli*; undercooked poultry can also harbour campylobacter – both cause food poisoning

- liver products: they contain too much vitamin A

- raw or runny eggs: they harbour salmonella

- seafood such as raw fish, oysters, prawns and other shellfish (unless cooked): they can also harbour salmonella and campylobacter.

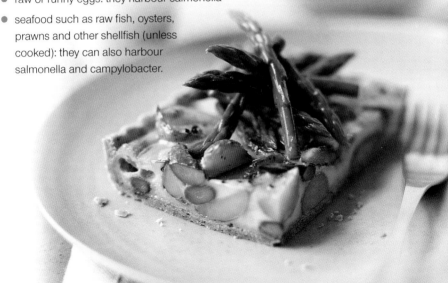

need to know . . . going nuts?

If you have a family history of allergies, asthma or eczema, the usual advice is to avoid eating peanuts during pregnancy. The idea is to prevent your baby becoming sensitized to peanuts before birth. This is the best available advice on the subject at the time of writing, though future research could change that.

ALCOHOL

Heavy consumption of alcohol by a pregnant woman is dangerous for her unborn baby, but there is a lot of debate about social drinking. Although there is scant evidence that one, two or even three drinks a week can harm, many mums play it safe and follow current government advice to avoid drinking alcohol altogether during pregnancy.

CIGARETTES

On this subject there is no debate: smoking in pregnancy robs your baby of oxygen. It raises the risk of miscarriage, premature labour and of having a small sickly baby. Giving up is worth every effort.

MEDICINES AND OTHER DRUGS

Many drugs cross the placenta to reach your baby. In general, a baby is most at risk in the first three months of gestation, but some drugs can harm at any stage. Always check with your pharmacist, midwife or doctor before using an over-the-counter drug. Similar cautions apply to complementary therapies, including aromatherapy.

Street drugs, as you can imagine, are even more dangerous. If you are a user, do your baby a favour and get specialist help.

If you are on long-term medication, for instance for diabetes or epilepsy, it may need to be changed during pregnancy. But don't stop it without medical advice.

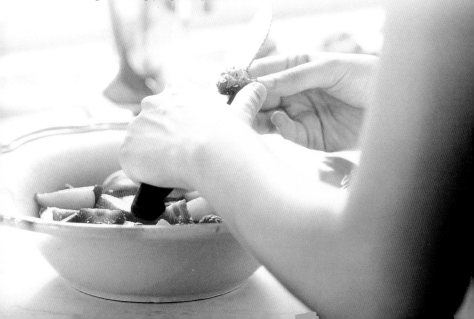

SUPPLEMENTS

Folic acid, a B-vitamin, helps to prevent spina bifida and other 'neural-tube' defects, as well as cleft palate (hare lip). That is why women should take a supplement of 400mcg folic acid daily, ideally from before conception until thirteen weeks.

EXERCISE

- Regular exercise helps to alleviate constipation and other discomforts of pregnancy. It may also help to shorten labour and make birth easier.

- You can usually continue with your favourite exercise, except for contact sports, but don't take up strenuous new activities.

- Drink enough water and avoid getting overheated, which might be harmful to your baby.

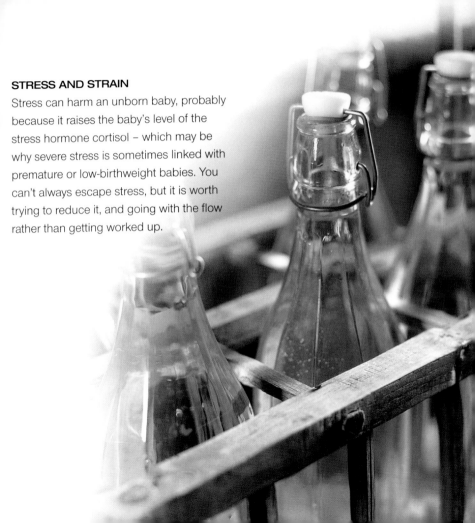

STRESS AND STRAIN

Stress can harm an unborn baby, probably
because it raises the baby's level of the
stress hormone cortisol – which may be
why severe stress is sometimes linked with
premature or low-birthweight babies. You
can't always escape stress, but it is worth
trying to reduce it, and going with the flow
rather than getting worked up.

EARLY DAYS

The first trimester – up to and including week twelve

Appearances are deceptive. There is not much to see on the outside during the early months, but inside your womb your baby is really taking shape. It is no wonder that you feel exhausted for so much of the time.

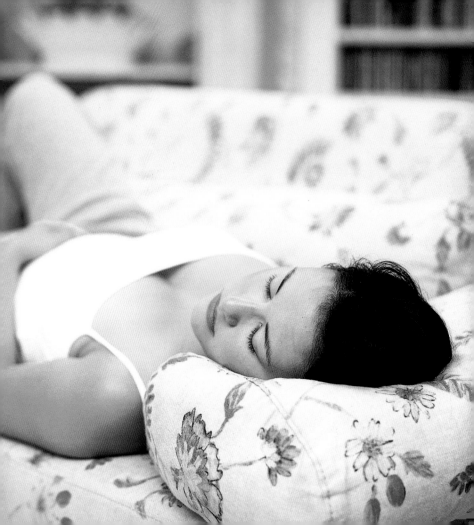

week three

The story starts at week three, because at week one you're not even pregnant. Pregnancies are dated from **the first day of the** mother's **last** menstrual **period**. But conception usually occurs about two weeks later – that's when some **300 million sperm try speed-dating**, and the winner joins up with your ovum (that's your egg).

By week three, the **fertilized ovum** has started to burrow into the wall of the uterus. It is also **dividing rapidly**. By the time it implants into the womb, it's already made of about 200 cells. And it has begun to divide into **two parts**; the inner part will become your **baby**, while the outer part will become your baby's life-support machine in the form of the **placenta**.

week four

Now your ovaries produce more **progesterone**. This hormone stops the lining of the uterus shedding, and throwing the baby out with it.

Meanwhile your **tastes change**. You could go off coffee. Or you may have a metallic taste in your mouth.

the real deal . . . on cat trays and gardening

If you've got a cat, you now have the perfect excuse to get someone else to clean out the litter tray. Cat poop contains the parasite toxoplasma, which is potentially harmful to your baby. If you have a garden, you can't legislate for passing animals using it as a loo, so either wear gloves when gardening or, even better, lounge around decoratively sipping a cool drink while someone else works up a sweat.

your baby

Your little embryo is a little disc about the **size of a match-head**, and made up of three distinct layers.

- The outermost layer is called the **ectoderm**, and will become your baby's brain, nerves and skin.
- The inner layer, or **endoderm**, will develop into organs such as the lungs, liver and gut.
- The middle layer, called the **mesoderm**, becomes bones and muscles.

Over the next few weeks, these three simple biscuit layers will fold and refold many times to form all the intricacies that make a human being. The process kicks off during week five, when the disc folds into a cylinder and also forms a head and a tail. At this stage, your baby is about **1.5mm long**.

your body

Around now, you may get some lower abdominal pressure, which feels exactly like the start of a period. It is nothing to worry about. The cause is simply that your pelvic organs are congested.

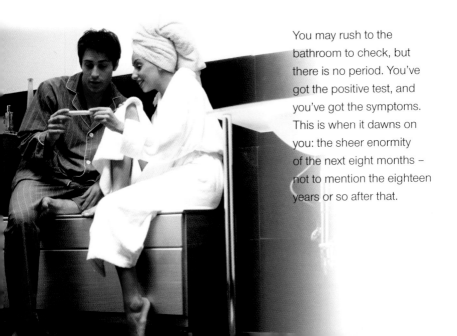

You may rush to the bathroom to check, but there is no period. You've got the positive test, and you've got the symptoms. This is when it dawns on you: the sheer enormity of the next eight months – not to mention the eighteen years or so after that.

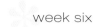

the inside story

Your baby embryo has a distinct curve. With her tail, she looks a bit like a **seahorse**, but without the snout.

The complex folding of the tube of ectoderm begins. This eventually becomes the **brain and nervous system**. At one end, the bulge of **brain** is already forming.

On the face, the **eyes and ears** are just tiny pits.

There are no limbs yet, only two pairs of **buds**, upper and lower.

By the end of this week, your baby's length from her head to her bottom (called **crown–rump length** or CR length) is about **4mm**.

the real deal . . . morning sickness

It's called morning sickness because doctors (especially those who don't have children) think it goes away before lunch. Not true. It can last all day – and it's made worse by strong smells and by movement (such as travelling on a bus).

The reason for morning sickness is the hormone HCG, made by the placenta. Levels of HCG tend to be higher if your baby is thriving, so take it in your stride if you can.

- Eat little and often.
- Ginger can help – try adding fresh ginger to stir-fries, ginger tea, even ginger biscuits.
- Acupressure wristbands can work too.
- If you can't keep anything down, speak to your doctor. Tablets can be prescribed for severe morning sickness.

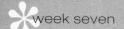

the inside story

By now, your baby already has a **heart** with four chambers that beats about 150 times a minute.

The **sex organs** are formed, though the testicles aren't external yet.

His arms and legs look like miniature paddles, and soon they will make tiny movements. But he can't control his limbs, and you can't even feel any movement. This isn't surprising since in total your baby is only **5mm long** – barely bigger than a mung bean.

need to know . . . miscarriage

Sadly, the loss of a baby before twenty-four weeks is common. It's often said that twenty per cent of pregnancies miscarry, but research shows it's much more common because women can miscarry early on, before they know they are pregnant.

- Symptoms include pain and bleeding. If bleeding doesn't stop of its own accord, you may need to have your womb evacuated, either under general anaesthetic or using drugs.
- In most cases, a miscarriage has no known cause. Many women blame themselves and wonder if it could have been prevented. But the vast majority of miscarriages are inevitable. The process just seems to be nature's somewhat ruthless way of eliminating imperfect babies.
- Having one miscarriage doesn't mean that you will have another. But if you have three or more miscarriages, you will need tests to rule out a treatable blood disorder.

the inside story

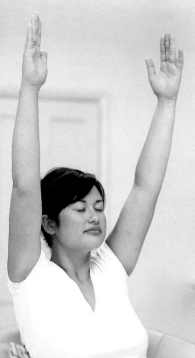

Now your tiny embryo is **9–10mm** long. She looks less like a baby seahorse and more like **a little human**.

If you could see her, her **skin** would appear **transparent**, with blood vessels threading beneath it.

Her **upper lip** is formed, and she has bumps that will become her ears.

Her **limbs** are longer and becoming limb-shaped, with elbows and wrists. Her **fingers** and **toes** are webbed; the fingers lose their webbing before the toes.

Her **eyes** are on the sides of her head, like a fish – which is appropriate, considering her aquatic existence.

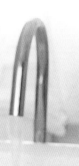

need to know . . . symptoms

- Headache caused by hormonal changes is common in the first trimester. Try to avoid tiredness and dehydration. If you need to take something, the occasional paracetamol is usually safe.

- Constipation is caused by the hormone progesterone. Ease it by eating more fruit and vegetables, and taking regular exercise.

- Breast tenderness and enlargement are usual. The better the baby is doing, the more sensitive your breasts may become.

- Vaginal discharge is common, because your vagina and cervix are congested and produce more mucus. However, if there's itching or a smelly discharge, see your doctor.

- Tiredness can be extreme. If you can't carry on, relax in a nice warm (not hot) bath.

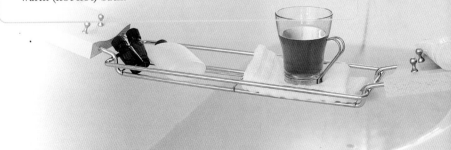

the inside story

Your baby's **back is straighter** and the 'tail' that was there at week six has vanished. This week he grows up to **3cm** (crown–rump length).

Your baby's **eyelids** almost cover his eyes now.

His **jaw** is formed, and there's a new bump on his face – his **nose**.

Little touch pads form at the ends of the fingers.

> If you haven't been given an appointment to see your midwife yet, now is the time to make one.

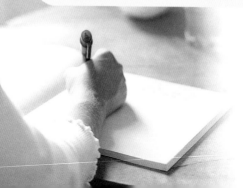

need to know . . . twins

There are two kinds of twins. Identical twins develop when a fertilized egg splits into two early on, while non-identical twins come from two separate eggs. The non-identical kind can be a boy and a girl, and are no more alike genetically than any other two siblings.

- Identical twins are around a third as common as their non-identical counterparts.
- If you're having twins, your early pregnancy symptoms, especially morning sickness, can be a lot worse. Your bump becomes visible sooner too.
- Twin pregnancies are often more complicated, with a higher risk of pre-eclampsia and of premature labour. Your womb was designed for single occupancy, so growth can be restricted – that's why you'll get frequent scans. With some identical twins, there's also a risk of a potentially serious condition known as twin-to-twin transfusion syndrome.
- As if to make up for all this bother, twins can be twice as much joy after they're born.

antenatal drill

Your first **antenatal** appointment, called a 'booking' appointment, is a long session. The **midwife** takes your medical, personal and family history. You get info on **scans** and other tests, and **healthy living advice**.

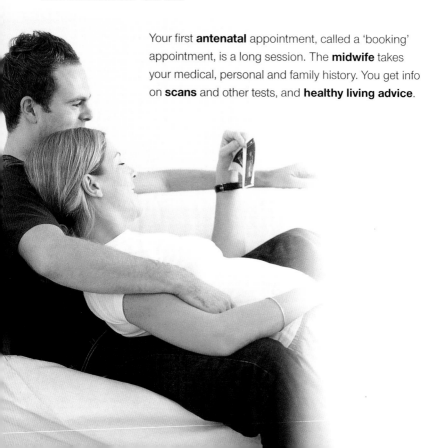

At booking, or soon afterwards, there's a **blood test** for **anaemia**, for **blood grouping** and to rule out hepatitis B and sexually transmitted infections, all of which can affect your baby. An HIV test is on offer too.

At every appointment from now on, your **blood pressure** and **urine** are checked and your **abdomen** is examined. At intervals there are more blood tests and scans to consider – for instance, another test for anaemia at twenty-eight weeks.

need to know . . . your first scan

Scans use high-frequency soundwaves to build up a picture. Although it may be fuzzy, your baby's general shape and beating heart are both easily visible.

The first scan is at ten to thirteen weeks. Its main purpose is to check that your baby's size matches what would be expected from the date of your last period. In about fifteen per cent of cases, the due date is adjusted after this scan. The other purpose of the scan is to check if your baby's bringing a pal.

In most hospitals, you can buy a photo of your baby's scan. If you want it for posterity, photocopy it or scan it into your computer, because thermal images fade.

the inside story

Your baby **weighs about 8g** and she is only **5cm long** (crown–rump length). Yet she is a miniature masterpiece because all her **vital organs** are there: brain, lungs, kidneys, liver and bowels.

Your baby has separate **fingers**. Most of her **joints are formed**, and she moves a lot, in a random way.

While you've been busy at the clinic, your baby has been busy developing apace. Officially she's no longer an embryo – she's a fetus, meaning 'little one'.

need to know . . . antenatal tests

The most common tests are designed to screen for Down's syndrome and for spina bifida (and related defects). You are likely to be offered an AFP (alpha-fetoprotein blood test) for spina bifida at around sixteen weeks, but the exact timetable of tests on offer depends on where you live.

Screening tests are 'non-invasive' but do no more than reveal the probability of your baby having a particular problem. All pregnant women are now offered screening for Down's syndrome such as blood tests and/or a scan of the back of your baby's neck (nuchal lucency). CVS (chorionic villus sampling) and amniocentesis can give a definite diagnosis, but they are invasive procedures.

Discuss the tests with your midwife and decide which, if any, you want. It is better to think the process through before testing rather than after you get the results.

the inside story

Your baby is growing fast. Despite weighing only **14g**, he is somehow **chunkier**. His bones are thicker and harder, and he is **6cm long** (crown–rump length) – about the size of a **kiwi fruit**.

The **placenta** is completely formed, though, like your baby, it continues to grow.

WHEN TO GO ON AIR

Maybe you are bursting to share the news. On the other hand, isn't it lovely to keep the secret of the baby growing inside you?

The end of the first trimester is a good time to start going public. For one thing, you too will soon look chunkier, as your womb rises out of the pelvis, and your bump will soon show.

For another thing, the risk of miscarriage drops significantly after thirteen weeks, so it feels safer to tell the world. It is your decision.

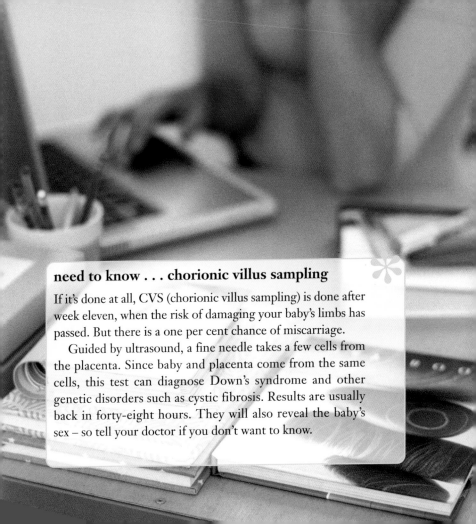

need to know . . . chorionic villus sampling

If it's done at all, CVS (chorionic villus sampling) is done after week eleven, when the risk of damaging your baby's limbs has passed. But there is a one per cent chance of miscarriage.

Guided by ultrasound, a fine needle takes a few cells from the placenta. Since baby and placenta come from the same cells, this test can diagnose Down's syndrome and other genetic disorders such as cystic fibrosis. Results are usually back in forty-eight hours. They will also reveal the baby's sex – so tell your doctor if you don't want to know.

THE MARVELLOUS MIDDLE MONTHS

The second trimester – thirteen to twenty-seven weeks

This is a time of rapid growth for your baby – and for you. As your bump becomes obvious, you may get friendly smiles from complete strangers. You are probably looking and feeling blooming during these three months, so make the most of it.

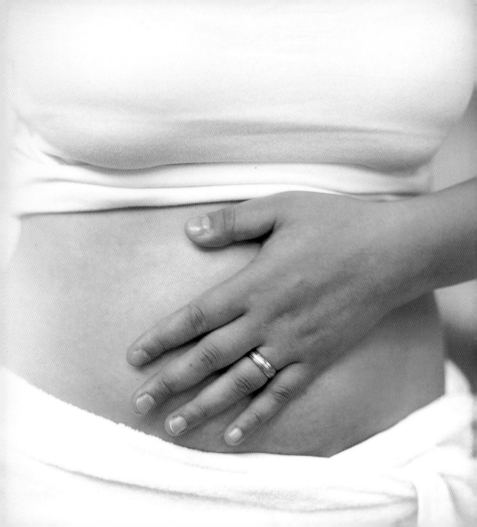

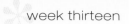

your baby

Now your baby is **7.5cm** long and weighs around **20g**. She has got little **nails**, and she looks like a miniature baby, albeit only **the size of a peach**. Her neck is developing, so she can move her head better now. And she makes more **facial movements** too, including opening and closing her mouth.

your body

Your **uterus** (or, rather, its top part, the bit medics call the fundus) can probably just **be felt** above the pelvis.

You can stop taking folic acid supplements since all **your baby's organs are formed**, though they are not quite the finished product yet.

Morning sickness may ease around now, and soon you will have that **pregnancy bloom** that poetic types rave about.

need to know . . . your antenatal records

If you are curious about all those medical abbreviations, here is what some of them mean:

LMP last menstrual period

EDD estimated date of delivery

BP blood pressure

FBC full blood count (blood test)

MSU mid-stream urine (sample)

GTT glucose tolerance test (a series of blood tests for diabetes)

NAD no abnormality detected

VE vaginal examination

FMF fetal movements felt

FHH fetal heart heard (with either a Doppler machine or a fetal stethoscope)

NE not engaged (meaning that the widest part of your baby's head is still above the brim of your pelvis)

USS ultrasound scan

BPD biparietal diameter (the size of your baby's head estimated by USS).

the inside story

Your baby is now **8–9cm long** and a whopping **25g in weight**.

His brain and nervous system have not yet made connections with his muscles, so his **movements** are still **random and reflex** in nature, but there are plenty of them. He is practically **a gymnast**.

Your baby's kidneys are actively making urine now, which he wees into **the amniotic fluid** that surrounds him in the womb. If you are wondering where that goes – he swallows it again.

Genitals are developing fast, and **a baby boy's penis** will soon be **obvious on a scan**. If you don't want to know your baby's gender, ask the ultrasound radiographer to keep quiet about it.

need to know . . . boy or girl?

- All a woman's eggs carry one X chromosome. If an X-carrying sperm fertilized your ovum, you are having a girl (XX), while if a Y-carrying sperm fertilized your ovum, you are having a boy (XY).

- More boys are born than girls, though precisely why is a mystery. There are just as many sperm carrying X chromosomes as there are carrying Y chromosomes.

- Ovaries or testicles start developing around nine weeks. By twenty weeks, they are well-developed.

- If you have a boy, his penis may be visible on a scan from around thirteen weeks, but his testicles lie hidden inside his belly until thirty weeks.

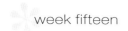

your baby

Your baby is now **10cm long** and weighs about **50g**. She is about the size of **an orange**, only much more interesting.

Now she has a decidedly human face and a neck. Her **eyes** are even becoming **sensitive to light**, which she can discern through the skin of your belly.

If you could see your baby, her skin would be transparent, apart from **a fine downy growth of hair**, called lanugo, over her body and head.

Her bones are still mostly cartilage, though calcium is accumulating within them, helping them to harden into **real bone**. As your baby's **muscles** develop, she moves her thin arms and legs, although you can't feel this yet. She tries out **lots of movements**.

your body

Your **skin** is likely to feel **smooth** and **nicely hydrated**, though you could develop more moles and freckles, or even larger patches of **pigmentation** on your face. These patches are called chloasma, and they often fade after your baby's born. If you notice anything unusual, check with your midwife or GP.

cover up

The sun accentuates any pregnancy-induced pigmentation, so wearing sunscreen is essential. The lighter skinned you are, the more you need it. A wide-brimmed hat is useful too; together with loose floaty clothes, it can be a sexy look.

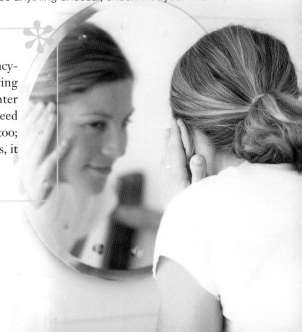

the inside story

Your baby is **growing fast** and his legs are getting a lot longer. Suddenly he is **80g in weight**.

His ears are almost totally developed, so **he can hear your voice**.

Importantly, his brain cells now link up with his spinal cord and from there to his muscles. That's why his **movements** begin to be **more coordinated**. Some, like hiccups, are still involuntary.

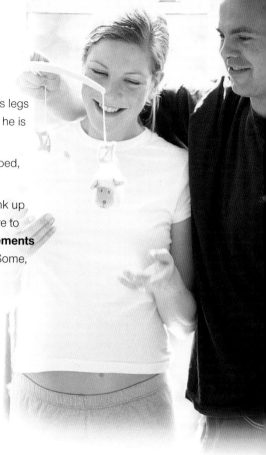

need to know . . . amniocentesis

- Amniocentesis means drawing off a sample of amniotic fluid, along with some cells shed by your baby. There are more of these cells after sixteen weeks, when amnio is done.

- Like CVS, this test is done under ultrasound control.

- The risk of miscarriage is usually under one per cent.

- You will be offered amniocentesis if one of your screening tests turns out positive, or if there is some other reason for thinking your baby might be at risk of a chromosome (genetic) disorder. This could be anything from sickle cell disease to Down's syndrome.

- In some cases, amnio is used to diagnose infections before birth or to assess how well a baby's lungs have developed.

- The cells gathered in an amniocentesis must be grown in the laboratory before the chromosomes are analysed, so results can take three weeks. However, newer laboratory techniques can give quicker results.

your baby

Now your little one is about **12cm** long – about the size of an average avocado – and weighs **100g**. She gets plenty of nourishment via the **placenta**, but she doesn't yet have much fat on her. So while she has been getting longer, **her face looks lean**.

However, she has some hair on top, and she's got **eyebrows and even eyelashes**.

She uses her exquisitely formed features to try out different expressions.

Her ribcage is busy too, because she's **practising breathing movements**, though she is 'breathing' amniotic fluid, not air.

All in all, this is a very active time. It won't be long until you will be able **to feel her moving**.

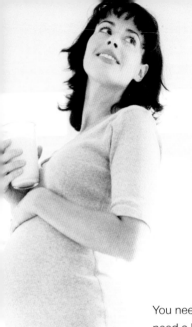

your body

With all the progress your baby is making, no wonder **your jeans are straining at the seams**. You need looser clothes around now, or you may opt to move straight into maternity wear. There is a huge range of **mum-to-be clobber** out there – so there's bound to be something to suit your lifestyle and your pocket.

You needn't get a nursing bra just yet but you do need a bigger size of bra than normal, and it must be supportive, so **a bra-fitting is a must**. In fact you will probably go up a size or two several times in pregnancy. If you are usually **a cleavage-free zone**, prepare for appreciative looks.

the inside story

Your baby is now **150g** and about **13cm long**. Fat is beginning to be deposited in all the right places, so that by the time he's born he'll be **the image of cuteness**. Some of this is 'brown fat', which works like an insulating blanket **to keep him warm** after he's born.

Now that his **fingerprints** are taking shape, he will be unique too. Even identical twins have different fingerprints.

He is very active physically, and may even have his own **diurnal rhythm** (unfortunately, this will not necessarily be the same as yours).

Deep inside his brain, a part called the thalamus has developed. This means that he can probably **feel pain** from now on.

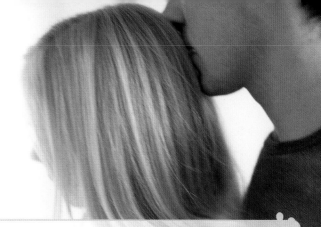

the real deal . . . emotional swings and roundabouts

Preparing to have a baby involves a great deal more than having antenatal checks and wearing a floral tent. You need to adjust emotionally too. At this time there is often emotional muddle anyway, thanks to a cauldron of pregnancy hormones. You may feel it's doing your head in.

Are you a cool calm office manager or a competent professional in your other life? Even so, watching the news on television could make you blub.

Pregnancy is a natural state, but for many women it is also a time of extreme highs and lows.

- Go with the flow and don't be hard on yourself.
- If you've got relationship issues, address these as calmly as you can.
- Tell your midwife about any serious worries or if you feel depressed.

the inside story

Your baby is now some **14cm** long and weighs **200g**, and there's another **200g** or so in there – the placenta.

Your baby has been in the womb for a while, but in fact she has served only **half her term**. To protect her tender body for the remaining weeks, glands in her skin now produce a thick greasy white gunk called vernix caseosa. This forms **a waterproof shield** that any cross-channel swimmer would covet, and it will still be there at birth.

Around now, **nipples** begin to show.

Deep within her jaws, **tooth buds** are beginning to sprout, for both her milk teeth and her permanent teeth.

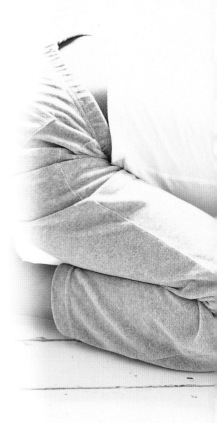

the real deal . . . the athlete within

Swimming movements, kicking, punching – your baby does them all. It is only around now that you become aware of his movements. At first, they feel like vague flutterings, a bit like wind. But at some time between twenty and twenty-four weeks you will be in no doubt that your baby is on the move.

He may produce more kicks at night. This isn't because he is trying to be a nuisance. It is probably because your muscles are more relaxed then, so there is more space to move.

Many mums-to-be count the kicks, but there is no need to do so. However, if you notice that your baby suddenly becomes still for a few hours or more, tell your midwife without delay.

the inside story

Now **your bump** reaches up about 20cm above your pelvis. The little person inside is **15cm long** (crown–rump length), roughly the size of a premium **mango**. If there were any scales in there, he would tip them at **260g** or so. He is actually **bigger than the placenta**.

He has better body control, and can make **purposeful movements**.

And he can hear well, including **the sound of your voice** and any music that's playing. Loud noise makes him jump.

His heartbeat is now strong enough for your midwife to hear it with **a stethoscope** (the fetal kind that looks like a small megaphone). His **heartbeat varies** according to what is happening outside.

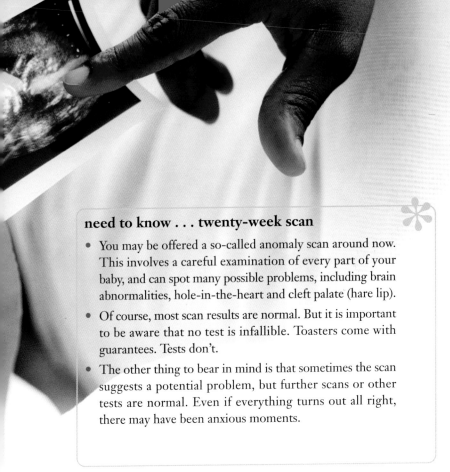

need to know ... twenty-week scan

- You may be offered a so-called anomaly scan around now. This involves a careful examination of every part of your baby, and can spot many possible problems, including brain abnormalities, hole-in-the-heart and cleft palate (hare lip).

- Of course, most scan results are normal. But it is important to be aware that no test is infallible. Toasters come with guarantees. Tests don't.

- The other thing to bear in mind is that sometimes the scan suggests a potential problem, but further scans or other tests are normal. Even if everything turns out all right, there may have been anxious moments.

your baby

Your baby's now about **300g** in weight and **16cm** long.

When she swallows amniotic fluid, her **taste buds** get tiny traces of the foods that you have eaten.

Her **intestines** are processing this, so there is already some waste in her bowel.

Although her **eyelids are still shut,** she can probably make out light and dark.

Her **memory is developing** too, so her experiences have a lasting impact. By the time she is born, she will be familiar with **the sound of your voice,** and the foods that you usually eat – this may help with breastfeeding.

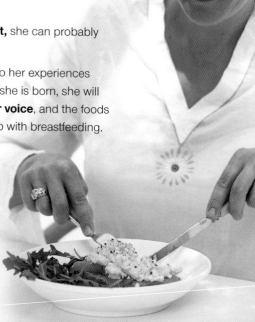

your body

Although you have probably gained only a few kilos, **your body is definitely changing**. You feel different and may look voluptuous. By now, your **bump is growing higher** by about 1cm a week. This rate continues until about thirty-six weeks.

need to know . . . placenta praevia

- A placenta that lies in the lower part of the womb is called a placenta praevia. In extreme cases, it can cover the inside of the cervix. In such a case, you would need a caesarean section to avoid possible fatal bleeding during labour.

- If an earlier scan suggested a low-lying placenta, you will have further scans to monitor this.

- The good news is that a low placenta can rise as the pregnancy progresses, making a normal birth possible.

the inside story

Now your baby is **19cm** long and weighs **350g** or so. Sweat glands have developed, and the rest of him is active too. His **brain is growing rapidly**, and the number of cells is actually increasing.

Boy babies have **a few primitive sperm** at this stage, while girl babies have around **six million eggs**.

As well as kicking and punching, your baby rolls around, crosses and uncrosses his legs, and reaches out. He even **sucks his thumb**.

Sometimes he moves less. That is because he has a distinct **sleeping–waking cycle**, which you will become attuned to. Research shows that babies even **dream in the womb**, but probably about nothing much. Before birth there are not many experiences on which to base interesting dreams.

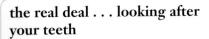

the real deal . . . looking after your teeth

One effect of the hormone oestrogen is that your gums may look swollen and could bleed. This usually happens when brushing, though you could also find blood on your lips on waking up in the mornings.

- Don't stop brushing, but use a softer toothbrush than usual.

- Floss if you know how to. But be careful: floss is like a cheese-wire. It is worse to floss badly than not to floss at all.

- During pregnancy, see your dentist for a check-up. In a few months' time, you will probably be too busy.

the inside story

Your baby weighs about **450g**. She is **20cm** long (crown–rump length), but there is **half a litre of amniotic fluid** for her to stretch in. Feeling her move can be an intense **bonding experience**.

Her **skin is still wrinkly** because there is not much fat, but it is already four layers thick. And the lanugo hair is getting darker now.

Her eyes are still closed. Buts **she hears really well**, and begins to know the voice she hears most – yours.

Her lungs may be immature, but that doesn't stop her practising **breathing movements**.

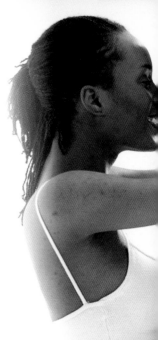

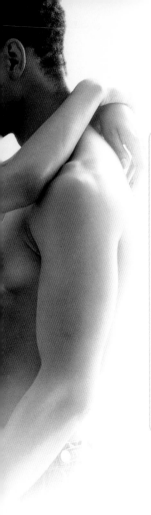

the real deal . . . sex in pregnancy

Some pregnant women are really keen, while for others sex is the last thing on their mind. For your partner, your shape may be a turn-on or he may worry about hurting the baby.

Your baby can hear you now, and he may also become particularly active after sex. But there is no need to worry about 'doing it in front of the children'.

Unless you have bleeding, placenta praevia, or other complications, sex does no harm, and you can continue well into the third trimester. By then your bump can get in the way, so you may want to explore different positions. Lying on your side, either as 'spoons' or . . . oh, just enjoy finding out for yourselves.

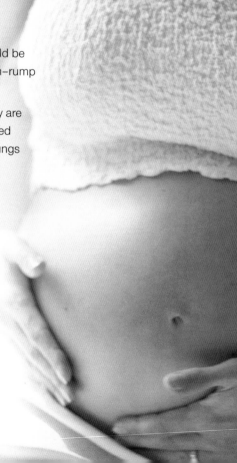

your baby

If your baby arrived this week, he would be a tiny human measuring **21cm** (crown–rump length) and weighing around **550g**.

His **lungs are still immature**, but they are starting to make **a vital chemical** called surfactant, which helps air enter the lungs after he's born. With expert help, your baby could probably survive now.

your body

But you may wonder how **you will survive** the next sixteen weeks if your baby stays put. By now, you may be **tired**, breathless after exertion and **lacking in 'zip'**. That's because your heart is working forty per cent harder than before your pregnancy. Try to **rest with your feet up** during the day. If you feel extra-tired, tell your midwife; you could be **anaemic**.

the real deal . . . work

Many women start their maternity leave at around thirty weeks, but some work longer, preferring to have more leave after the birth. It depends on how well you and your baby are, and on the work you do. Heavy lifting, prolonged standing, long hours and shiftwork are all potential hazards to your baby. So are toxic chemicals and some infections.

Your employer should allow you to change your duties and/or hours if there is a risk to you or your baby. If that's impossible, you may need to start your leave early. If you can't reach an amicable agreement, contact the Maternity Alliance, your trades union if you have one, and/or your midwife or GP.

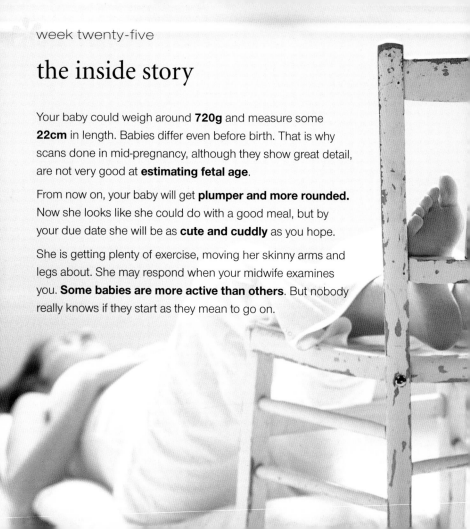

the inside story

Your baby could weigh around **720g** and measure some **22cm** in length. Babies differ even before birth. That is why scans done in mid-pregnancy, although they show great detail, are not very good at **estimating fetal age**.

From now on, your baby will get **plumper and more rounded.** Now she looks like she could do with a good meal, but by your due date she will be as **cute and cuddly** as you hope.

She is getting plenty of exercise, moving her skinny arms and legs about. She may respond when your midwife examines you. **Some babies are more active than others**. But nobody really knows if they start as they mean to go on.

need to know . . . pre-eclampsia

Pre-eclampsia is a common but serious complication which comes on after twenty weeks. If the condition is severe, it can be life-threatening for you and your baby.

Pre-eclampsia is due to a placenta problem, and causes high blood pressure and protein in your urine.

Watch out too for:

- severe headaches
- blurred vision
- pain in the upper abdomen
- swelling of hands and feet

and tell your midwife if you have any of these.

However, you yourself cannot tell you've got pre-eclampsia, which is one good reason for having antenatal checks.

At the moment there is no known treatment for the condition, and your baby may need to be delivered early.

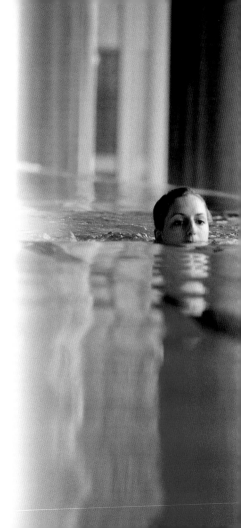

your baby

Now your baby is around **23cm** long and weighs about **950g**.

Inside his brain, his nerve cells begin to develop a coating of **myelin**. Part protein, part fat, myelin insulates a nerve and **helps it to conduct signals faster**. That is why your baby now has faster responses to sound, touch and bright light. He may even **sway in time to music**.

your body

Your bump reaches above your navel, but your brain is going south. If you are less mentally sharp than you were, there is a reason. Scans show that a woman's brain shrinks during pregnancy. While research isn't conclusive, it seems that brain size probably returns to normal afterwards.

Swimming is great exercise at almost any stage in pregnancy and can relieve anxiety as well as minor aches and pains. By now you will need a maternity swimsuit though.

---

need to know . . . twins

If you are expecting twins, you will probably find that you have many more minor symptoms of pregnancy, as well as lots more kicks to feel.

Until around twenty-eight weeks, twins often grow at the same rate as a single baby. After that, they are likely to grow more slowly. Scans are usually routine for twins at twenty-four, twenty-eight, thirty-two, thirty-four and thirty-six weeks.

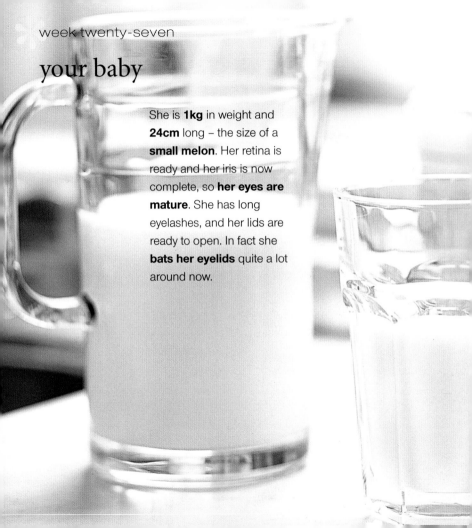

your baby

She is **1kg** in weight and **24cm** long – the size of a **small melon**. Her retina is ready and her iris is now complete, so **her eyes are mature**. She has long eyelashes, and her lids are ready to open. In fact she **bats her eyelids** quite a lot around now.

your body

Unwelcome symptoms can appear now, thanks to your growing baby and the hormone progesterone, which has a relaxant action on your gullet and blood vessels.

Heartburn, or indigestion, can occur at any stage in pregnancy, though it is sometimes worse as your waistline expands.

- Eat smaller meals and eat more often.
- Drink milk to help to neutralize stomach acid.
- Avoid spicy meals and eating late at night.

Piles can cause itching around the back passage, as well as a palpable lump, and even bright-red bleeding during a bowel action.

- Constipation can make things worse, so eat plenty of fruit and vegetables.
- Ask your pharmacist or GP about ointments or suppositories to ease the symptoms.

Varicose veins are similar to piles, but in a different place. You could get unsightly blue lumps or aching at the end of the day.

- Keep active.
- When standing, move from one leg to another to keep the muscles pumping.
- When sitting, put your feet up.
- Maternity support tights help.

THE HOME STRETCH

The third trimester – twenty-eight to forty-two weeks

During these final three months your baby's body gets
its finishing touches. As the weeks go by, you may
wish that he would hurry up and make an appearance,
so that you can have your body back to yourself.

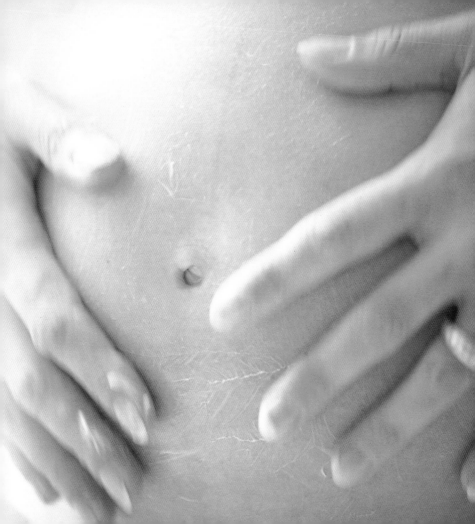

the inside story

Your baby is now **25cm** long (crown–rump length) and weighs **1.1kg**.

Vernix has developed all over. On the scalp, **fine hair is sprouting**, while on his body, lanugo hair starts to thin out.

If he is a boy, his **testicles** are now in his scrotum.

If you are having a girl, her **vagina** is completely formed, but her vulva has yet to develop fully.

need to know . . . rhesus disease

There are two main kinds of blood group – the ABO system and the rhesus system. If you are rhesus negative and your baby is rhesus positive, you could make antibodies against him. These can pass through the placenta and destroy his blood cells, making him anaemic.

Some good news: while some of your baby's cells can enter your circulation, the antibodies you make can't reach your baby in your first pregnancy. However, once you start making them, they can affect future pregnancies.

That is why, if you are rhesus negative, you will receive an injection of anti-D to clear your bloodstream of stray cells from your baby and prevent you making antibodies.

Anti-D is usually given at twenty-eight and thirty-four weeks, as well as after delivery.

It is also good practice to have an anti-D injection if you undergo any procedure (such as CVS or amniocentesis) that allows your baby's blood to enter your circulation.

your baby

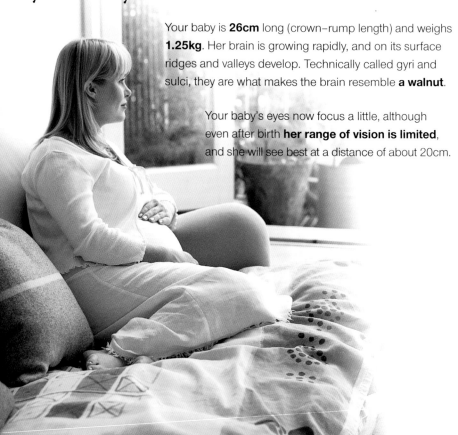

Your baby is **26cm** long (crown–rump length) and weighs **1.25kg**. Her brain is growing rapidly, and on its surface ridges and valleys develop. Technically called gyri and sulci, they are what makes the brain resemble **a walnut**.

Your baby's eyes now focus a little, although even after birth **her range of vision is limited**, and she will see best at a distance of about 20cm.

your body

Your **bump continues to rise** at a rate of about 1cm a week, but you haven't run out of belly space just yet.

Your breasts could feel extra-heavy from now on. A **sleep bra** at night will keep you more comfortable.

If you are waddling or have trouble keeping your balance, it's because your **centre of gravity** has changed. Wearing flatter shoes helps.

Rest with your feet up every afternoon. This also has the happy effect of increasing the placental blood flow, so **it's good for both of you**. If you are still working, arrange a break in the middle of the day to do this.

the real deal . . . antenatal classes

As D-day approaches, you may be apprehensive about what's to come. Now is the time to book antenatal classes. These address your physical well-being and help with emotional preparation too. The setting is informal, but they are classes in the sense that they are not to be missed.

your baby

Three-quarters of the way there, your baby is plumper now. He weighs around **1.4kg** and is **27cm** (crown–rump length). With his legs stretched out, he is more than **40cm** long.

Your baby is probably lying head down – the so-called vertex presentation. If he is in **the breech position**, or bottom down, he could still turn on his own until around thirty-six weeks. Your midwife can confirm which way he is lying.

Most often, **a baby keeps his head down** and his legs curled up, except when he's practising his boxing and football skills.

His lungs are not quite mature yet, because there is not enough surfactant (see page 60).

your body

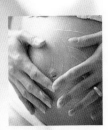

Garishly coloured (red or purplish) **lines could appear over your belly, upper thighs and even breasts**. Don't you wish you'd been smoothing on lotions and creams for the last few months? Well, don't worry. While rubbing on creams won't do any harm, these **potions probably won't do any good** either. It's the inbuilt resilience of your skin that determines whether you'll have **stretch marks** after the birth. Some women don't

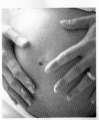

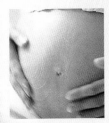

get them even if they carry twins and gain 30kg. If you haven't got any, you too are **blessed with the right genes**. If you have got them, rest assured that stretch marks eventually become **thin, white marks** that are far less obvious.

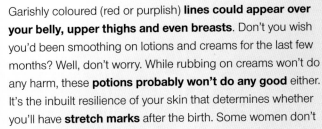

your baby

Now she's around **28cm** (crown–rump length) and weighs about **1.6kg**. Her skin is smoother because there is more fat under it.

In her lungs, the amount of **surfactant** surges, which helps her to breathe later.

She is now very active, and may move more at night. Her **brain is active too**, and is busy making more connections. As a result, she forms **memories**. You may want to talk to your baby, sing to her or **play her your favourite music**. She may not grow up to share your tastes, but it's nice to try.

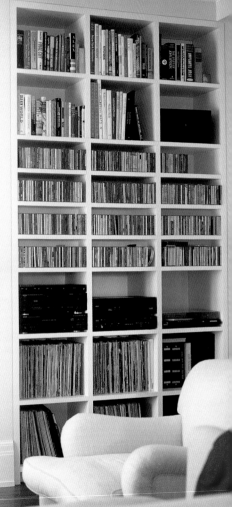

the real deal . . . emotional stuff

This bit is slightly scary, but there is no avoiding it. No matter how many books you read about having babies, you cannot really appreciate quite what it's like until it happens. A baby changes your life for ever – and it's not just a mum thing either, because babies alter dads too.

Your relationship with your partner shifts; it may become more stereotypical. The woman becomes a mother rather than just a lover or wife. The father often becomes the sole breadwinner, at least temporarily.

Life is more meaningful as well as more enjoyable, but it is also more serious because there is more at stake. It is worth discussing in advance the emotional, financial and practical adjustments you might both have to make.

your baby

Now your baby weighs **1.8kg** and is **29cm** in length (crown–rump length).

His face is increasingly expressive, and he sometimes **sticks his tongue out**. Within his confined quarters, he uses his senses, tasting amniotic fluid, listening intently, and **using visual clues** too.

While there is less room for him to move, if he is head down you will be very much aware of **his legs kicking near your ribs**.

He also touches his face and grabs his cord. You may even be able to **feel his fingernails** scratch harmlessly within you. If you have two babies in there, they are likely to be **alternately stroking and kicking** each other. That too is harmless.

your body

Your bloom could be **wilting** a little.

If you stand for long or lie on your back, you may feel faint because there is less blood returning to your heart. **Avoid standing for very long.** In bed, lie on your side to avoid the weight of your baby pressing on your large blood vessels.

Itchy skin can be **soothed with emollients**. If your palms or soles itch, your should tell your midwife since this could be a symptom of obstetric cholestasis. This rare but serious liver problem can begin with intense itching of hands and feet.

Braxton-Hicks contractions are practice contractions in preparation for the real thing. They are not painful, and they don't make the cervix dilate.

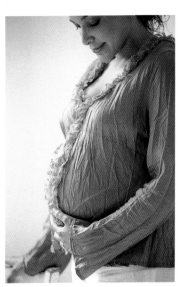

your baby

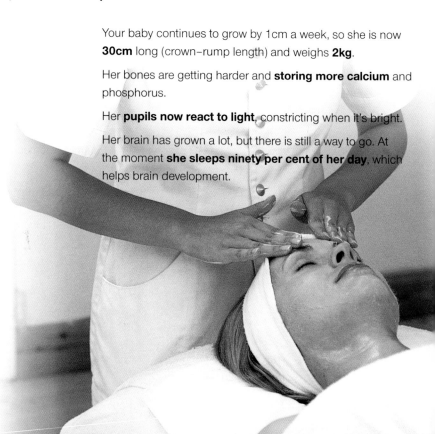

Your baby continues to grow by 1cm a week, so she is now **30cm** long (crown–rump length) and weighs **2kg**.

Her bones are getting harder and **storing more calcium** and phosphorus.

Her **pupils now react to light**, constricting when it's bright.

Her brain has grown a lot, but there is still a way to go. At the moment **she sleeps ninety per cent of her day**, which helps brain development.

your body

You have gained 9kg or more. Your baby and placenta are around half of this – **thanks to pregnancy hormones**, the rest is you. Your uterus alone weighs 800g, compared with 70g before pregnancy.

Your belly sometimes feels **tight**, especially if you walk or exert yourself. Take this as a hint to put your feet up.

If your baby is breech, you can **encourage him to turn** by spending time on all fours, with your head lower than your pelvis.

feel-good ideas

- Treat yourself to a manicure, pedicure or facial (make sure you mention that you are pregnant, as not all products are suitable).
- Go to the hairdresser's. Highlights are usually safe throughout pregnancy, but dyes that touch the scalp may not be.
- Consider an outing to a place that doesn't allow children, whether it's a cinema or a stately house. It will be harder later.

the inside story

Your baby now weighs **2.3kg**, and is about **32cm** long (crown–rump length). Fat makes up almost fifteen per cent of his body weight, so he already looks adorable.

Importantly, his **immune system** is maturing – which includes his lymph glands, spleen, tonsils and adenoids. Although he gets lots of **antibodies** from you through the umbilical cord, it is also important for him to have his own active immunity **to fight off infections** when he's born.

the real deal . . . nest-building

If you haven't felt the nesting instinct already, now is the time when you may get the urge to prepare the nursery, clear out cupboards, paint walls and so on. Your energy may be limited, and so may your time if your baby arrives early, which makes it unwise to embark on huge tiring projects. However, do think about acquiring essentials such as:

- cot and bedding
- baby clothes including stretch-suits, socks, vests, cardigans and bonnets
- nappies
- car seat
- pram or pushchair
- baby bath.

If you are superstitious, as many mothers-to-be are, you could simply source the things you'll need. Check out shops and online retailers. Either send your partner out later to get all the stuff or, if delivery times are suitably short, arrange to put in your final order at the last minute.

your baby

She is **33cm** long (crown–rump length) and weighs a little more than **2.5kg**.

The number of fat cells rises rapidly, especially around those cute shoulders. Her hair is up to **4cm** long, and either dark or fair.

There is less room to move, but there is still plenty of amniotic fluid. This **muffles most of the sounds** she hears, but your voice comes across loudly, as your baby can feel the **vibrations** as well as hear the sound.

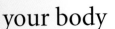

your body

The bump reaches up to the lower end of your breastbone, and you are wondering if you will ever **see your feet again**.

Now that your centre of gravity is much further forward, your **back may ache** in response to the strain. Swimming helps to relieve it, and it keeps you fit as well. To ease backache you can also get on the floor on all fours and **alternately stretch and arch your back like a cat**.

Passing urine frequently is common now, especially **if you stand a lot**. If you also have burning, tell your midwife; it could be an infection.

Leaking colostrum from your breasts can happen at almost any time, or not at all; both are normal. Whether you are leaking or not, get fitted for **a nursing bra** soon.

your baby

He weighs **2.75kg** and is **34cm** long (crown–rump length). If he held his legs out straight, he would be nearly **50cm**.

Now your baby spends more time **awake**. You could say he's getting to know you better. In fact, **he could be born at any time** between thirty-seven and forty-two weeks.

your body

Your belly may develop strange **bumps and lumps** as
your baby moves. He may still turn, but he is now unlikely
to change from a breech to a **vertex presentation**, since
there simply isn't much room to manoeuvre.

need to know . . . twins

- In the case of twins, thirty-seven weeks is considered full
  term. The average weight of twins is 2.5kg each, but they
  can be much lighter or much heavier. Boys are a bit
  heavier than girls. Identical twins are a bit lighter than
  non-identical (fraternal) twins.

- Even when twins arrive early, premature twins tend to
  do better than premature singletons.

- Since birth is more hazardous for twins, a woman having
  twins is more likely to have a caesarean. Some sixty per
  cent of twins are delivered this way. It depends a lot on
  how they are lying at term. If both twins are head-down
  (vertex), you could probably have a vaginal delivery unless
  the babies are premature or there are other problems.

your baby

Your baby's maturing is all but done now, except for her **lungs** and her **brain**. She is now **35cm** (crown–rump length) and weighs around **2.95kg**. It is often said that growth slows down in the last month or two, but in fact your baby is still putting on about **250g** a week.

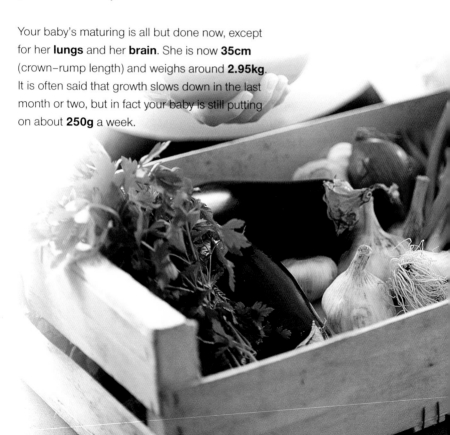

your body

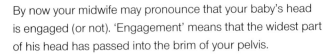

By now your midwife may pronounce that your baby's head is engaged (or not). 'Engagement' means that the widest part of his head has passed into the brim of your pelvis.

When this happens, your pelvis may feel a bit crowded, so you could need to pass urine more often.

It becomes harder to walk without waddling and almost impossible to sit down with your legs crossed. On the plus side, there is less pressure under your ribcage.

the real deal . . . a good idea or three

- If you don't get your groceries delivered, set this up. It will save you valuable time when your baby arrives.

- Think of names if you haven't already. This will avoid having to call your baby 'Junior' or 'Yellow Blanket' for two weeks until you and your partner can agree.

- Make sure your hospital bag is packed and left in an obvious place (see page 101). It is all too easy to leave it behind in the heat of the moment.

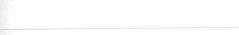

the inside story

Your baby is now **36cm** long (crown–rump length) and weighs **3.25kg**. He has been putting on fat and even has a bit of a pot-belly.

His head may be deep into your pelvis now.

He has **300 bones**, more than you have. That is because some of his baby bones fuse together as he grows.

His bowels are actively making **meconium**, a sticky dark-green substance made of dead cells, amniotic fluid and the **lanugo hair** that he has been shedding.

Meanwhile the placenta is gradually starting to fail, in readiness for your baby's reliance on **his next life-support system** – you.

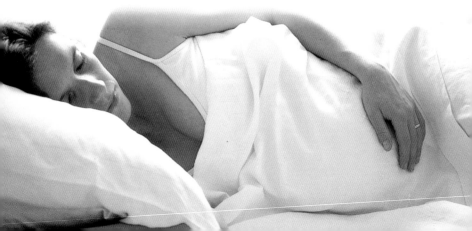

the real deal . . . insomnia

By now you may be finding it hard to get a good night's sleep. There are lots of possible reasons for this. Your bump is pretty big, so it is hard to get comfortable. And maybe you are lying awake wondering what it will all be like. The chances are that you are not getting much exercise in the day, so it is more difficult to nod off. Some women are also woken by vivid dreams, probably due to hormones.

Try:

- a warm milky drink
- relaxation exercises
- a pillow or two wedged under your belly to make you more comfortable.

If all else fails, simply lie still and rest. It is not the same as sleeping, but it's the next best thing.

your baby

She weighs around **3.4kg** and is about **37cm** long (crown–rump length).

Her immune system is maturing, so that she will be able **to fight off infections** in the world outside.

Inside her brain, **new connections** are forming.

Apart from that, she has not changed very much since last week. She is just **waiting in the wings**, somewhat squashed but still kicking. She passes the time by **sucking her thumb**, making faces, and practising her breathing and her reflexes.

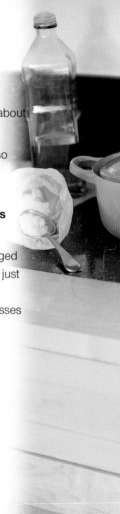

your body

The non-pregnant you is but **a distant memory**. You may be feeling massive and sluggish, both mentally and physically. **Don't be hard on yourself** – this is entirely normal.

If you feel the need to fill the time, **cook and freeze** a few meals for after the birth.

Make sure **your camera is ready** and fully charged so you don't get caught on the hop.

Actually, since babies turn up **exactly when it suits them**, it is probably better not to be ready. This could be the most effective way to ensure **a prompt arrival**.

need to know . . . your baby's heart rate

His heart makes 120–160 beats a minute. Some say that you can tell from the heart rate whether you are having a boy or a girl, but science shows you can't. However, your baby's heart rate does vary according to how active he is.

your baby

Now your baby is about **38cm** long (crown–rump length), weighs **3.5kg**, and is **ready to be born**.

His lanugo hair has almost gone.

He makes breathing movements, but it is only when he starts breathing air that his **heart and circulation will be fully mature**, with the left ventricle pumping out oxygen-rich blood, and the right ventricle sending oxygen-poor blood back to the lungs for a refill.

The placenta is only some fifteen per cent of **your baby's weight**.

His bowels are pretty full, so he will soon need a nappy.

Some women think they can hear **their baby cry in the womb**, but that's another myth. To make any sound with his **vocal cords**, he needs air.

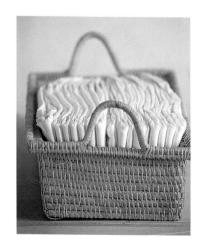

your body

You are likely to feel huge and impatient. It may seem pointless arranging anything to do, since **labour could begin at any moment**. However, the days can drag unless you have something planned. You can always cancel if necessary.

Most of the weight seems to be in the pelvis, **where the action's going to be**. By now you may have some diarrhoea and low-back pain.

Or you could get **a 'show'**. This is a pinkish or red discharge. Basically it is the mucus plug from your cervix, which drops out as your **cervix ripens and begins to dilate**. Contractions will follow – though how soon is anyone's guess.

So your baby's **overstayed her welcome**? It happens. In fact, it is absolutely normal for babies to arrive at any time two weeks before or after the official estimated date of delivery (EDD).

If you go significantly beyond your due date, you will be checked often to see all is well. This will include **listening to your baby's heartbeat** and a scan to assess the amount of amniotic fluid, which is a sign of **fetal well-being**.

By now, you have probably developed a resentment of being pregnant. Unfortunately, for many women, it is coupled with a horror of being **induced**.

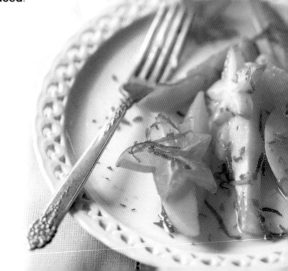

need to know . . . inducing labour

Labour tends to be riskier for both the baby and the mother if you are very overdue. That's why, if you haven't gone into labour by forty-two weeks, you are likely to have one of these:

- prostaglandin pessary
- rupture of your membranes
- oxytocin drip.

None of these methods is nearly as gruesome as its sounds. Even so, many women prefer to try natural methods such as:

- eating a hot curry
- driving on a bumpy road
- long walks
- sex
- nipple stimulation
- drinking raspberry leaf tea
- feasting on fresh pineapple (it contains an enzyme that may encourage contractions).

The only tactic that probably works is sex, largely because it provides a dollop of prostaglandins right where the midwife will soon put those pessaries. It is also more pleasant.

LABOUR & BIRTH

This is the most exciting and productive time of all – a tumult of hormones and action (your action, it is to be hoped, not that of the doctors). But, whichever way you deliver, it culminates in that magical moment when you finally hold your baby in your arms for the first time.

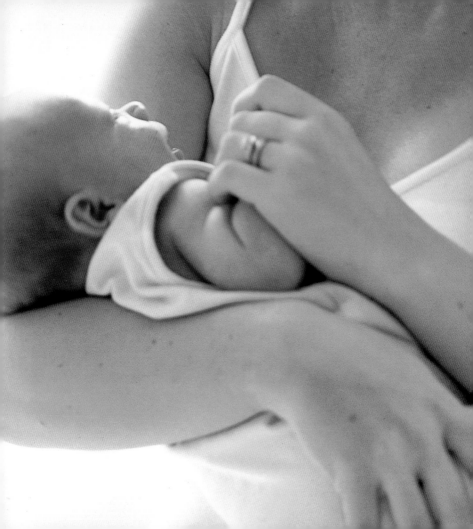

preparing for labour

In a sense, the past eight months, possibly even the past few years, have all been preparation for labour. But some specific things need a little thought.

BIRTH PLAN

A birth plan can incorporate religious or cultural preferences, as well as any other wishes about how you'd like things to go. Do you want to walk about in labour? To have a massage? To avoid intensive fetal monitoring or an episiotomy? To cut your own cord? To keep the placenta as a memento? Or to have an epidural as soon as you hit the labour suite?

Equipment such as a birthing pool needs to be organized in advance, not just jotted down in your birth plan. Whatever you decide, try to be flexible on the day, and allow deviation from the plan if you are given a good reason for it. Every labour is individual and, let's face it, what matters is that the experience is a healthy one for your baby.

HOSPITAL BAG

It makes sense to have a bag ready even if you are planning a home birth, since you could end up in hospital. Pack:

- toiletries for yourself
- nightdresses and dressing-gown
- nursing bra
- slippers
- maternity pads
- clothes and nappies for the baby
- bottled water
- snacks such as energy bars
- maybe some music to listen to
- a sponge for dabbing your forehead
- change for the pay-phone.

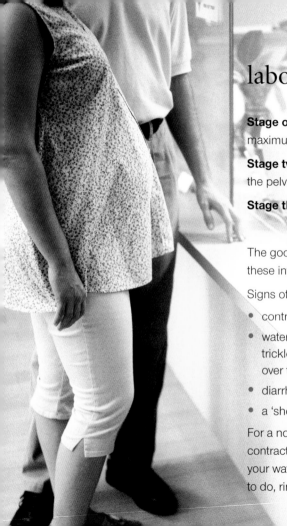

labour

Stage one is dilation of the cervix to a maximum of 10cm.

Stage two is your baby's descent through the pelvis and out into the world.

Stage three is delivery of the placenta.

The good news is that only the first two of these involve any real work on your part.

Signs of labour include:

- contractions, irregular to begin with
- waters 'breaking', sometimes as a trickle, sometimes in a flash flood all over the carpet
- diarrhoea or back pain
- a 'show'.

For a non-home birth, go to hospital if your contractions are regular and strong or if your waters break. If you are not sure what to do, ring your midwife or the labour ward.

PAIN

Pain is a very individual thing, as is what to do about it. You may find the pain worse than you imagined or not as bad. One thing to remember is that relieving pain helps you to feel in control of your labour. Discuss options with your midwife.

need to know . . . monitoring in labour

There are three main ways for medical staff to check on your baby's well-being:

- by listening to the heartbeat intermittently by means of a stethoscope or Doppler probe
- by external electronic monitoring via a belt on your belly, to record the baby's heartbeat and your contractions
- by fetal scalp monitoring; a tiny clip attached to the unborn baby's head gives an electronic readout of her heartbeat.

birth

At stage two, your contractions get longer and more intense, bringing the urge to bear down. Listen to your body, unless the midwife tells you to hold on. After a few intense pushes, your baby's head should be born. Once this happens, the rest of him follows swiftly, guided by your midwife's expert hands.

The dullest stage of labour is delivery of the placenta, but you still have some input. One option is an injection of an oxytocic drug into your leg. This makes your uterus contract, so the placenta separates. Your midwife then gently eases it out. The other option is to let nature take its course, which may mean heavier bleeding.

For some women, there is a fourth stage. If you've had a tear or an episiotomy, stitches are done under local anaesthetic (unless there is an epidural in place). The stitches dissolve in time, so don't need removal.

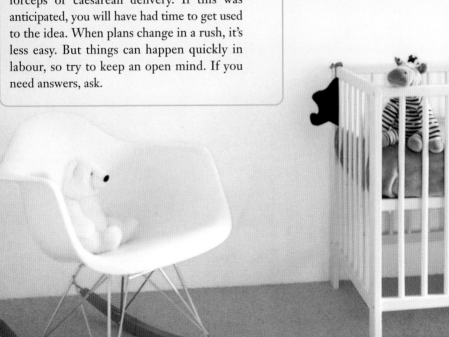

the real deal . . . not part of the plan

The 10cm trip down the pelvis is the most perilous journey a human ever makes. That is why babies sometimes need a ventouse, forceps or caesarean delivery. If this was anticipated, you will have had time to get used to the idea. When plans change in a rush, it's less easy. But things can happen quickly in labour, so try to keep an open mind. If you need answers, ask.

going home

So there you are, a bit sweaty and shaky perhaps, with your baby snuggled up on your breast, and tags on his ankle and wrist to remind you that he is all yours.

He is covered in vernix and a bit bloody too. His head may look squashed, depending on the labour. But in your eyes he is still the most beautiful thing you've ever seen.

Your midwife checks him (and you) immediately after the birth, and a junior paediatrician should also examine him top-to-toe before you both go home.

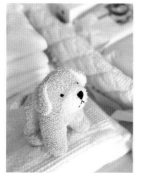

How long you stay in hospital depends on the delivery itself, how busy that maternity unit is, and what your home circumstances are. Nowadays a stay of six hours is almost the norm following a vaginal delivery, even for first-timers. In this almost indecent haste, it is easy to forget something. Make sure you get a cup of a tea and some toast. That humble refreshment is the very least you deserve.

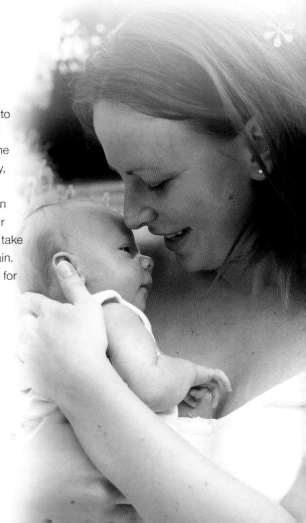

When you get home, don't try to do it all. In some cultures, new mothers don't lift a finger for the first six weeks after birth. Sadly, this custom is not part of the western way of life. But you can concentrate on being with your baby. Let the chores wait, and take every opportunity to get fit again. You need to be in good shape for your all-important new role.

useful addresses

Active Birth Centre
(antenatal and parenting classes)
25 Bickerton Road
London N19 5JT
020 7281 6760
www.activebirthcentre.com

Antenatal Results and Choices
(support and info on antenatal
tests and results)
73 Charlotte Street
London W1T 4PN
helpline 020 7631 0285
www.arc-uk.org

**Association for Improvements
in the Maternity Services** (advice
on parents' rights and choices)
helpline 0870 765 1433
www.aims.org.uk

BirthchoiceUK
(info on birth options)
www.birthchoiceuk.com

BLISS (the premature baby charity)
68 South Lambeth Road
London SW8 1RL
020 78209471
helpline 0500 618140
www.bliss.org.uk

**Caesarean Birth and VBAC
Information**
www.caesarean.org.uk

Group B Strep Support (charity
working towards the prevention of
group B streptococcal infections)
PO Box 203, Haywards Heath
West Sussex RH16 1GF
01444 416176
www.gbss.org.uk

La Leche League (advice and info
for women wanting to breastfeed)
PO Box 29, West Bridgford
Nottingham NG2 7NP
helpline 0845 1202918
www.laleche.org.uk

The Miscarriage Association
c/o Clayton Hospital
Northgate, Wakefield WF1 3JS
helpline 01924 200799
www.miscarriageassociation.org.uk

National Childbirth Trust (NCT)
Alexandra House
Oldham Terrace
London W3 6NH
0870 4448707
www.nctpregnancyandbabycare.com

**National Council for
One-Parent Families**
255 Kentish Town Road
London NW5 2LX
020 7428 5400
www.oneparentfamilies.org.uk

NHS Direct (info and advice
on health matters)
0845 4647
www.nhsdirect.nhs.uk

NHS Pregnancy Smoking Helpline
0800 1699169
www.gosmokefree.co.uk

Parents at Work (info on childcare
and employment rights)
1–3 Berry Street
London EC1V 0AA
020 7253 6253
www.parentsatwork.org.uk

SANDS (Stillbirth and Neonatal
Death Society)
28 Portland Place
London W1B 1LY
helpline 020 7436 5881
www.uk-sands.org

Tamba (Twins and Multiple
Births Association)
2 The Willows, Gardner Road
Guildford, Surrey GU1 4PG
0870 770 3305
helpline 0800 138 0509
www.tamba.org.uk

Women's Aid Federation (help for
women threatened by violence)
helpline 0808 2000247
www.womensaid.org.uk

index

picture credits

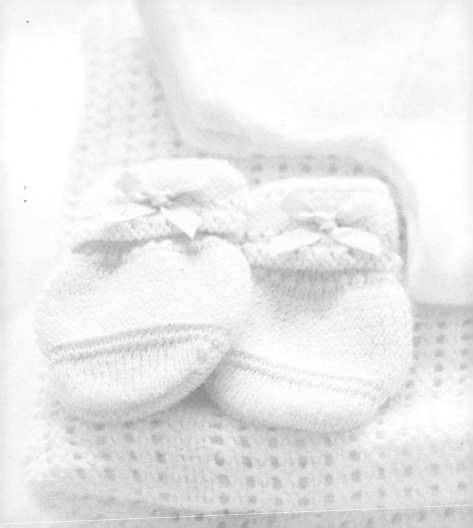